ACING THE FOURTH TRIMESTER

Dr. Talya Miron-Shatz and the Buddy&Soul team

INTRODUCTION: WELCOME TO ACING THE FOURTH TRIMESTER

It is a universally acknowledged truth that much like a Jane Austen novel ends with a wedding, once you give birth and go home with a baby you end up at home with a new baby.

And experience pure bliss.

Now, back to reality. Considering that you're still hormonal and bleeding, possibly recovering from surgery or stitching, and your baby basically is a fetus with a vocal range that suddenly carries, it's not surprising that the first three months after birth are referred to as the "fourth trimester." Unfortunately, the books, websites, and apps seem to stop after three; those that *do* discuss the first year, focus almost solely on the newborn. Once the baby's out you're no longer a part of the pregnancy community, but you're not quite a part of the parenting fold, either. And you're certainly not back to your old self – with sleep, habits, stress, anything and everything that a tiny creature can and will throw off (but aren't they cute?).

That's where we come in. Join us to learn how to juggle this time of emotional ups and downs, of changing relationships, habits, and priorities. No matter how your baby came into the world, you're indisputably handling a lot more than you used to. We'll provide you with the tools you need to ace the fourth trimester, making your postnatal adjustment smoother, easier, and more enjoyable.

There are three goals that we had in mind while creating this book. We want you to

1. Process your birth experience, whether it was positive, negative, or somewhere in the middle,
2. Learn strategies to help ease the difficult parts of your fourth trimester,
3. Help you create a post-birth roadmap to get you back to you.

If you're about to become a new mom (regardless of what number birth this is for you), you've certainly been exposed to the only two socially accepted options for your post-birth experience: You can either cuddle your eternally calm infant in the ethereal morning light on crisp white sheets, or you can (try to) nurse a screaming baby in your underpants and a spit-up splattered tee while your very own Eeyore-style raincloud hovers above. Naturally, social media and pop culture tells you that the two options are mutually exclusive. If you enjoy your infant, you're lying. If you are overwhelmed, you don't love your baby enough.

As you probably know, it's more complex than social media and pop culture would have you believe. Maybe you're feeling helpless with your newborn, annoyed at your partner, guilty over not spending enough time with your older children, stumped by chores that used to be easy habits, and overwhelmed by new responsibilities piled atop the old. And this isn't even to mention the physical recovery, which isn't negligible even in the best of case-scenario, considering you just ejected a future-voter from your swimsuit area.

But amidst all this coping, there is a middle-ground to be found, one that is happy and dirty, in control of all the moving pieces of your new life even if somewhat dazed by all of it. It's harder to depict in stock photos, sure. But you can build your own roadmap to navigate the post-birth landscape.

The fourth trimester will be stressful. It's not the time to begin training for the Ironman Triathlon or to submit your digs to *Better Homes and Gardens*. So drop your expectations, cut yourself some slack, and dare to enjoy this whole new crazy and unknown reality you are a part of. We can help you get there, by giving you the tools you need to process your birth experience, to identify and face your particular challenges, and to make sure that this birth only serves to boost your sense of you, rather than diminish it.

Remember, you just made a person. Acing the fourth trimester? Easy peasy.

It is important to keep in mind:

1. Even if you've already had a child (or several children), each time is new and different, and finds you in a different place in life.
2. All new beginnings are hard, and this is the mother of new beginnings (pun intended)!
3. Embrace your newness as a mom.

YOUR JOURNEY TO ACING THE FOURTH TRIMESTER

HOW TO USE THIS BOOK TO ACE YOUR FOURTH TRIMESTER

In this book you'll find ten great strategies for achieving the goals we listed above. You'll also find inspiring content and exercises you can engage with to help you ace your fourth trimester.

You will get the most out of this book by going through the strategies and associated exercises one by one. Of course, you can also simply read it the whole way through. But we recommend using this book by going through it in order, watching the TED talks, and doing the exercises. We have found the best way to do the exercises is by dedicating a notebook as your course journal. If you're reading this book on a PC, feel free to create a text file and use that as your course journal. Or you could simply use a good ol' pen and paper to do the exercises. Either way, we recommend keeping some method of writing handy while you go through the exercises in this book to optimize what you get out of it.

To maximize your experience with the Buddy and Soul book, share your thoughts and insights with us on social media! Post pictures relating to your progress on Instagram and Twitter, tagging @Buddy_N_Soul, and Facebook @Buddy&Soul.   By sharing with us on social media, not only can you help others with their personal journeys, you can read about those facing similar challenges.

Direct message us YOUR story @Buddy_N_Soul on Instagram and be anonymously featured for a chance to **win a Buddy&Soul three month free membership**.

If you really want to go all the way, visit our website, BuddynSoul.com, and explore all that we have to offer beyond 'Acing the Fourth Trimester'. In fact, we have three other books in the Pregnancy series that we think you might benefit from: Relationship Saver During Pregnancy, Sticking to Your Pregnancy Plan, and Loving Your Pregnant Body.

I'm Dr. Talya Miron-Shatz, CEO of Buddy&Soul, where Acing the Fourth Trimester and many more e-courses and books come from. I have a PhD in psychology and was very fortunate to do my post-doc at Princeton University with Nobel Laureate Daniel Kahneman. I've also taught at the Wharton Business School, University of Pennsylvania. Now I'm a professor at the Ono Academic College, and a visiting researcher at Cambridge University. I used to study happiness, and for a long time now, I've been studying medical decision making and helping organizations support people on their way to joy and health. One thing

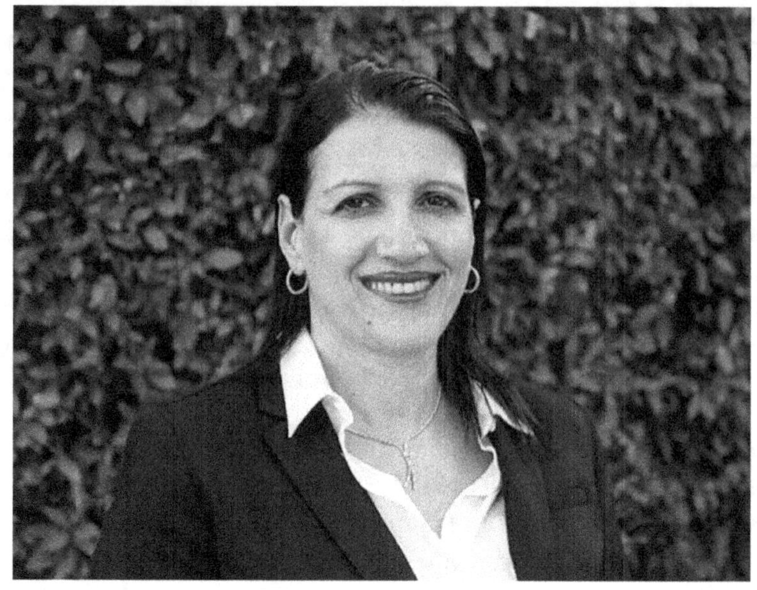

that struck me as unfair was that we were expecting people to change their life for good but weren't giving them the tools to do so. People deserve all the help they can get when breaking out of old patterns and moving their lives forward.

This is what Buddy&Soul does.

We support you in many ways by providing science-based actionable ways to sustain your body and mind. We help you sleep better, spark a change in your eating habits, and manage stress. We teach you how to create new habits and how to engage your willpower. We help you grow, claim your self-esteem, cultivate authenticity, reframe your life story, achieve your goals and so much more. Including Acing the Fourth Trimester. This one is particularly special for me, as I still remember myself being a new mom, feeling like my life has turned into a snow globe that someone just gave a good shake, then placed on its head.

We created unique course clusters for people dealing with specific challenges: students, patients, and pregnant women.

Everything you need to change your life for good.

I want to hear from YOU! Please feel free to send me an email with your thoughts, suggestions, and feedback regarding this book to talya@buddynsoul.com. I would love to hear what you think about this book and how it helped you with acing your fourth trimester. Your feedback is extremely valuable and will allow us to help more individuals, like yourself, to obtain the necessary tools and support needed to change their lives for good.

What's your biggest fourth trimester challenge?

Everyone has challenges in their fourth trimester, usually several. What is the biggest challenge you're facing? What the one thing you wish you could get under control?

1. My baby won't stop eating. I'm essentially wearing him as a necklace, and I feel my value as a person has been reduced to how much milk I can produce in a 24-hour period.
2. My daughter doesn't sleep in spurts longer than 45 minutes, and as a result neither do I. I'm a frazzled mess.
3. My baby is perfect, but even the most angelic being upsets the delicate ecosystem my family has established. Everyone has a new role now, and that takes getting used to.
4. Intimacy. My partner and I don't have time to be together, between the kids, the baby, and the demands of work and maintaining a household.

What are some of the challenges you are facing?

5. ____

6. ____

7. ____

Imagine that every time you had a Pap smear you were expected to form a gripping, *detailed* narrative to tell and retell to anyone who asked or even hinted at the test. And what's more, there are rules you *must* follow. Your story should be angsty, but not melodramatic; you should be the focus, but don't make it all about you; and regardless of how suspenseful it is or how unfavorable the outcome, it must have a happy ending. Any other result is shameful, and shouldn't really be discussed.

Now just lie back and relax, right?

According to Della Pollock's book *Telling Bodies Performing Birth: Everyday Narratives of Childbirth,* this is the exact dilemma many women are faced with when they're about to or have just given birth. They're unwittingly made part of a community that on the one hand values grotesque narratives, but makes any kind of failure a shame; your story should end with you feeling like a truly fulfilled woman, bursting with joy, love, and gratitude.

So where does that leave you? Do you tell your story, playing into the drama-gore-trauma narrative community? Do you play the role of fulfillment, to satisfy the audience? Or do you remain silent, and just deny that this pretty big, inherently feminine event had any real impact on you?

None of these are very good options, and in his doctoral dissertation, "The telling of childbirth stories," Anjani A. Soparkar points out what's missing. He posits that the **abundance of intimate physical details of childbirth stories fools us all into thinking we're hearing an intimate story.** But the intimacy of childbirth isn't in how dilated you became how quickly, or how many stitches you needed after the fact. **The true intimacy, the one you don't share, is in the psychological effect that birth had on you as a mother**.

We tend to shroud our stories in all those other details in order to reinforce the reality and the magnitude of what just happened.

Let's try and do that and really access what this birth—and the changes it entails—means to you.

EXERCISE

Which of the following images best captures your emotional memory of childbirth?
In what way? Write about the image in your journal and explain why. Take some time
brainstorming in your journal about your experience with Acing the Fourth Trimester
and then share your story with the Buddy and Soul community! Tag us on Instagram
and Twitter @Buddy_N_Soul, using the #BuddynSoulExpecting. By sharing with us on social
media, not only can you help others with their personal journeys, you can read about those
facing similar challenges.

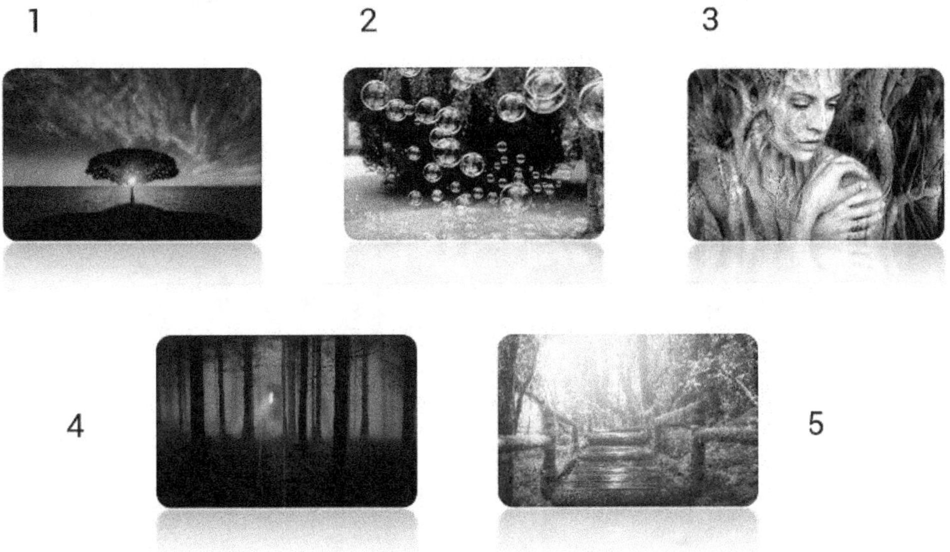

TIPS

Tip 1: Remember, there's no wrong way to experience childbirth. But if you feel this is too
difficult or painful for you, please consider speaking to someone (a friend or a professional)
who can help you process your experiences.

Tip 2: Having a hard time? Try instead to write out your birth story using no physical details,
and describing only the emotions that accompanied each stage.

Whose support do you find helpful in the fourth trimester?

We all need support in the fourth trimester. Who was your most helpful resource when you needed it?

1. My mom. She's always been my rock.
2. My spouse/partner. Because we're in this together.
3. An older friend. She's gone through this and knows what I need without asking.
4. A younger friend. She has less on her plate and is always willing to help out.
5. A Professional, such as a therapist or lactation consultant. I pay for the best and get the best.

Who else?

6. ____

7. ____

8. ____

6 "birth story" habits you should avoid

However you experience your birth—it's legit. There's no wrong way to go about doing one of the most momentous things a human body is capable of. However, there are a few bad habits you should avoid when constructing your birth story.

1. Don't make it a competition. If someone is telling you're their own birth story, try to listen and be empathetic, rather than reconstructing your own story to make it more dramatic, frightening, or topical.
2. Don't oversell it. In some communities there's an unspoken rule that if your birth wasn't dramatic, it hardly even counts. Don't fall for that trap. It's more than okay to have a positive experience, it's desirable! So don't be tempted to change the narrative of what happened to suit what someone else thinks is "acceptable."
3. Read the room. You're about to share something that is intensely important to you, but may not be to everyone else. So don't tell (or retell!) something that is deeply personal with people who may not care to hear it, or know how to respond properly. Don't put a piece of yourself out there just to get trampled.

Can you think of any others to avoid?

4. ____

5. ____

6. ____

Do I even need to "process" the birth of my child?

So-called "processing" seems like a millennial thing that's been invented to make women feel special. Did our mothers or grandmothers "process" their births? Isn't it just something that happens, and then you move on?

For:

1. Processing doesn't necessarily mean you need to create an insta post, or a piece of abstract art. It just means you need to acknowledge what you went through.
2. Birth is something BIG. Maybe the biggest thing a person can do, physically-speaking. It's worth taking the time to measure how you feel about just having done it.
3. Just because millennials do it, doesn't mean it's wrong.

Add your own:

4. ____

Against:

1. It's just another way to seek attention, after pregnancy is over and you're no longer the visible center of everyone's interest.
2. Whatever happened, happened. Good or bad, you need to be like Elsa and just let it go.
3. If it was good, there's not much to process. If it was bad, why focus on it? It seems like a lose-lose situation.

Add your own:

4. ____

DRIVING THE MESSAGE HOME

I'm glad that you've decided to start your journey towards Acing the Fourth Trimester. Each session of our course consists of a warm up talk followed by a hands-on component where you'll learn a new skill or idea and have a chance to start putting it into action.

We're going to start the Acing the Fourth Trimester book by taking a look at storytelling.

In the talk you're about to watch, Tyler Cowen examines the possible pitfalls of constructing and telling your birth story.

We think you'll find that the more you put into the course, the more you'll get out of it. So take full advantage of all our features and find your place in a community of people facing similar challenges.

Watch 'Be Suspicious of Stories' presented by Tyler Cowen at TEDxMidAtlantic on YouTube

Why telling my birth story is hard

There are pitfalls we are sometimes unaware of when it comes to constructing a narrative about our own lives, and this is especially true when constructing a story about a momentous occasion like giving birth. What was your pitfall? What made it difficult or tricky for you to tell the story of your birth? Write about it in your journal.

Direct message us YOUR story @Buddy_N_Soul on Instagram and be anonymously featured for a chance to **win a Buddy&Soul three month free membership.**

STRATEGY 2: Let go of the third-trimester regrets

Life is made up of a series of choices, and we often get stuck with regrets of abandoned possibilities. The road not taken often seduces us with limitless possibilities of what could have been.

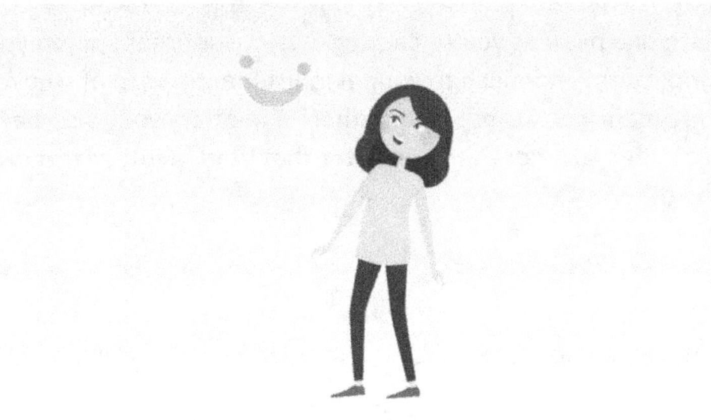

It could be the lack of proper preparation for birth, a natural water-birth that was abandoned for an epidural when the pain became too much, a surprise c-section you didn't think you needed, or the inner Hulk you channeled at innocent hospital staff who were just trying their best to help you. Regrets can form over any choice you make, big or small, and even over things you actually had no choice in, at all.

Luckily, there are a few ways to reframe regrets, and you need to find which works best for you:

The first is by neutralizing the glamour of the what-if-universe. For example, a newly postnatal mom might regret that she forgot to play her carefully curated playlist during labor. But who said it would be soothing, in real time? Maybe instead of making the pain more bearable, it would poison songs she loves with the pain-filled memories of childbirth. Maybe if you'd prepared all those frozen meals like you wanted, you'd have arrived at the delivery room too exhausted for the hours of labor ahead of you. There's simply no way of knowing.

The second way to reframe regrets is outlined by Dr. Hamilton Beazley in his book *No Regrets: A Ten-Step Program for Living in the Present and Leaving the Past Behind*. He recommends a powerful way to reframe your past regrets, by finding a lesson to be learned from them (*No Regrets*, p. 127). For example, I regret going to a particular hospital; I was warned that the staff there was rude and inconsiderate, but I went anyway and suffered a rude and inconsiderate staff. I may wish I had acted differently, but I can still learn a few things from it, like heeding others' advice even when I think I know better.

The third way to reframe regrets is by appreciating the circumstances that surround them. For instance, I regret not insisting on a vaginal birth when the staff recommended a c-section. There is no takeaway for the future here, the "damage" is done, and I'm not getting a do-over. But even so, I can still reframe. I didn't speak up because I was in unspeakable pain, confusion, and worry. I shouldn't underestimate that. Additionally, the pain of not having spoken up taught me that I truly care about having my voice heard, and that is a value I can pass down to my child, even if I can't act on it 100% of the time.

If regrets make us feel out of control, and like a powerless and sometimes foolish victim in our own life, reframing them gives us that control back. We can nullify the power of our regrets, and they can fade.

Living with regrets can be a heavy burden. Our shoulda-coulda-wouldas taint the present, instead of informing it. But **we can come to terms with our regrets, without denying or minimizing them**, by reframing them.

EXERCISE

Step 1: Late one night as you're packing away your breast-pump you happen to touch it in a particular pattern, and much to your astonishment a wisp of smoke forms itself into a magical Pregnancy and Labor Godmother. She offers you to go back in time and **change one element of your labor or third trimester that you deeply regret**. **What would you wish had happened differently?**

Write your answer in your journal.

Step 2: Alas, the magic wears off at the twelfth wail of a newborn's cry. But **you can still reframe it, using one of the three techniques** we've learned. Try it out in your journal!

How do you neutralize the glamour?

What lesson can you learn from this event?

What can you appreciate about the situation?

Write your answer in your journal.

TIPS

Tip 1: True, you can't change the past. But you can change how you relate to it, by releasing your regrets and 'what if's.

Tip 2: For that extra cathartic edge, you can take a pen and paper, and write out all your regrets and 'what if's. Tear that paper into pieces, and feel yourself releasing your regrets. Share your now-released regrets by snapping and uploading a photo of the paper shreds! Share your victory picture with the Buddy and Soul community! Tag us on Instagram and Twitter @Buddy_N_Soul, using the #BuddynSoulExpecting. By sharing with us on social media, not only can you help others with their personal journeys, you can read about those facing similar challenges.

Tip 3: For more on letting go of regrets, check out our course, Declutter Your Mind. 

10 Reasons it's beneficial to 'what if' your third trimester regrets

With the enormity of childbirth behind us, we suddenly have the time to wonder if we did everything right getting here. Regrets surrounding pregnancy and birth can be an unwanted burden, and it might be useful to try and explore the what-if universe to help alleviate it. Here are some reasons why.

1. Some 'what if's are not only in the past, and if you feel they are right for you, you might be able to act on them now. What if I had started working out a few times a week after I gave birth? Instead of wondering - get your gym clothes on and go for a run!
2. Use this as an opportunity to help your friends get a different perspective on things, and avoid similar regrets: *What if I had done better research into the birth center?* might help others make a more informed decision when they face a similar choice.
3. Don't make the same mistake twice, right? Thinking back to your regrets might help you understand yourself better, and help you avoid similar situations in the future.
4. Regrets are a part of life, and you need to allow them to become a part of *your* life. This doesn't mean you should sit around all day wondering 'what if;' but it's okay to say, "I regret that" rather than trying to avoid thinking about the situation altogether.
5. The paths you choose in life made you the person you are today, and it is completely normal to wonder 'what if' you'd have chosen a different path. These 'what if's are a part of the natural course of life, it would be crazy to assume they wouldn't pop up in your head from time to time.
6. Oftentimes, if you follow a 'what if' trail of thought, you'll realize that's not a path you'd have wanted for yourself, after all: What if I'd have had the home birth I wanted and planned for, but then something went wrong? Sticking to my plan wouldn't have been for the best.
7. Some of the best experiences and relationships came out of regrets and situations that we might have faced differently, if we could go back. You might not have stood up to that hateful midwife who said, "You think this hurts? Just wait!" but it made you ever-so-appreciative when the shift changed and the sweetest nurse came on to deliver your baby. Acknowledging this might help you let go of the annoyance that you have linked to your 'what if's.

Add your own:

8. ____

9. ____

10. ____

Which of the following traits help you most with releasing your regrets?

There are many traits that can help you let go of your regrets. Which do you feel will help you most with releasing them?

1. Decisive. When I make up my mind to do something, I rarely change it back. If I decided to go to a particular hospital, I made that choice for a reason.
2. Enthusiastic. I'm excited to try new things, and if they don't work out the way I planned, I'll know for next time.
3. Patient. I don't need to see results immediately. If experts think it will pay off in the long run, I'm willing to play the long game.
4. Efficient. I like to do things once, correctly. This seems like the best way of making peace with my past, changing how I experience things, and breaking patterns.
5. Rational. It may sound like an elaborate system of lying to myself, but it's one backed by proper scientific research. I don't know exactly how airplanes work, either, but I'm on board with both.

Add your own:

6. ____

7. ____

8. ____

The positive lesson from my negative regret

Regrets are interesting in that, if left alone, they have a half-life of *never*. They can pop up even years down the road, leaving you wondering if you did the right thing, chose the right doctor, really needed that emergency c-section... That's why it's better not to leave them alone, but to try and learn from them. How did you learn from your regret, and control it instead of letting it control you? Take a few moments to write about this in your journal.

Direct message us YOUR story @Buddy_N_Soul on Instagram and be anonymously featured for a chance to **win a Buddy&Soul three month free membership.**

I often ask myself- "what if I had chosen differently? What would my life look like now?" These seem to be questions we all ask ourselves rather often, wondering what different paths we could have taken and where would we be now had we chosen differently.

The following section addresses regrets and what ifs. Regrets can consume us, or we can look at them as lessons for life and find ways to become at peace with them. In the following video Kathryn Shulz talks about regrets, and why it is important to not-regret them, using her tattoo as an example. Watching her will hopefully prepare you for letting go of your lingering third-trimester regrets, and maybe provide ideas on how to accept your regrets and what ifs so you can make the most of your fourth.

Watch 'Don't Regret Regret' presented by Kathryn Schulz on YouTube.

How releasing regrets helped me be more positive

Sometimes the weight of regrets is such that you don't even notice it's there, until it's gone. Suddenly, everything in life seems a shade or two lighter. Write in your journal about how releasing your regrets helped you to be more positive and feel better about various aspects of giving birth and your life afterwards.

Direct message us YOUR story @Buddy_N_Soul on Instagram and be anonymously featured for a chance to **win a Buddy&Soul three month free membership.**

<u>STRATEGY 3: Pinpoint your Fourth Trimester challenges</u>

The long-anticipated event is finally here. You've just given birth to your precious new baby. You've gotten to hold him (or her) in your arms, little fingers have already clutched yours. You've brought your baby home to his new nursery, and maybe he's met his older siblings. And then challenges begin.

Physically, you might be adjusting to new sleeping patterns (or lack thereof), recovering from a caesarean or an episiotomy, nursing unsuccessfully, nursing successfully (engorgement, meet mastitis; you two will be rooming together for the next several months), or dealing with the baby blues (as real as any physical struggle). Emotionally, you might be feeling hormonal (but woe beside the person who dares say this to you), weepy, insecure, or lonely. Maybe you're not feeling attached to your child, or you're feeling guilty over instant attachment to this baby, when you didn't with the older ones. And then you experience some external challenges, like juggling more than one child, a colicky baby, a hovering mother-in-law with An Opinion, feeling smothered by the abundance of visitors, or starved for social interactions with people whom you didn't birth yourself.

Maybe one of these suggestions rings true to you. Maybe several do. Maybe none do. No matter what your challenges are, let's figure them out. **The most important element of being a good mom is taking proper care of yourself first.** Airport security videos don't lie, after all, and you need that metaphoric oxygen mask on yourself before you can help anyone else. And the first step towards taking care of yourself is identifying just how you are feeling and **what your challenges are** now that you are postnatal. Remember, everyone has challenges with a new baby. And the more aware you are of your challenges, the more you will be able to challenge them right back. So take the time to ask a question you may not have had the time or presence of mind to consider – how am I doing?

EXERCISE

Step 1: Use your journal to **make a list of your postnatal challenges now**. Try to think of physical, emotional, and "external" challenges that may be hindering you.

Step 2: **Write out possible ideas to help relieve some of the pressures** that are piling up.

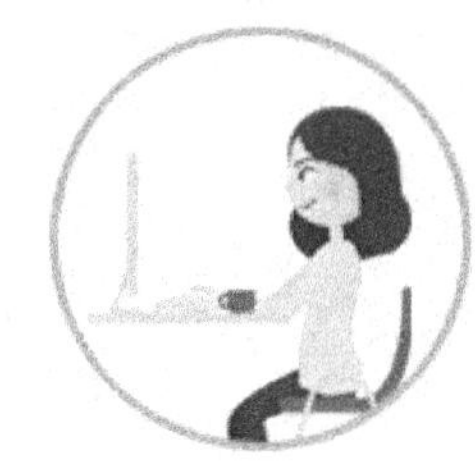

TIPS

Tip 1: Don't judge yourself harshly. Every mom has challenges afterbirth.

Tip 2: Try to be as specific as possible. This way you'll be better at articulating your challenges.

Tip 3: Not everyone has a mother who is able or willing to help (or whose form of help is welcome), so be creative: paid help, cutting standards, deciding to let the baby cry while you have a breather, or take-out meals are all viable options.

I've read all the books, will I even have any fourth trimester challenges?

Challenges are for those types who are under-aware. I, however, will have nothing to worry about, because, well I'm super aware of my capabilities, and I planned in advance for any deficits I may have. I know what to expect, and I'm ready for anything.

For:

1. Awareness means you'll recognize the challenge in real time, not that you won't have to face it.
2. Challenges can come from the outside, and not only from the inside (meaning, there are things beyond our range of control). You may have planned for the most challenging birth experience imaginable, but until you actually face it, there's no knowing how you'll do.
3. Your challenge might be how to deal with people who can't accept that you're acing the mom-thing. Do you shout them down? Do you keep correcting them? Challenges don't mean you're failing, they mean you've come in contact with another point of view. And trust us, there are plenty of those around.
4. Challenges are good! They help me grow.

Add your own:

5. ____

Against:

1. Challenges are a direct result of a lack of awareness. If you plan, you simply cannot be challenged.
2. This isn't my first rodeo. I know what to expect. I'm not bragging, but this parenting thing is something I happen to be prepared for.
3. I've micro-managed myself down to the last detail. There's no room left for challenges.

Add your own:

4. ____

7 Tips for finding your fourth trimester challenges

For some, finding their postnatal challenges is easier than saying their ABC's. For others, however, the challenges may be hiding under various guises, like "I should be able to do this," or "this just is what it is." Here are some helpful tips that can help you discern what some of your challenges are.

1. Think categorically: physical challenges, emotional challenges, baby-related challenges, mom-related challenges, etc.
2. Approach challenges from a non-judgmental place; you'd be surprised how lack of judgement can help your true feelings float to the surface!
3. Be real. As opposed to the face you put on for others, you don't have to be embarrassed of admitting to yourself that something is hard for you.
4. Imagine you are preparing a dear friend for childbirth: what would you tell her to look out for, the one thing no one likes to talk about?

Can you think of any tips?

5. ____

6. ____

7. ____

My biggest post-natal challenge

Discussing your challenges is not only beneficial for you, but it can also help other mothers out there know that they're not alone. Write in your journal about your biggest postnatal challenge and know that you're not alone!

Direct message us YOUR story @Buddy_N_Soul on Instagram and be anonymously featured for a chance to **win a Buddy&Soul three month free membership.**

We're going to continue the Acing the Forth Trimester book by taking a fundamental look at some of your postnatal challenges.

In the TED talk you're about to watch, Jennifer Senior shares her expertise at the growing anxiety and pressure placed upon new parents today. Nowadays there is tons of literature on how to raise your kid in exactly the best way possible, almost all of it contradictory, of course. All these how to's are completely overwhelming, and crisis inducing. I use the word crisis, because studies are showing that crisis is the common parental experience nowadays after having a baby. We take on an incredible amount of responsibility to raise our children to be happy, healthy, and successful. All this pressure can start from day one, really impacting your postnatal period and what you are feeling now.

Watch 'For Parents, Happiness is a Very High Bar' presented by Jennifer Senior on YouTube.

10 Normal postnatal feelings according to Senior

In Jennifer Senior's TED Talk, *For parents, happiness is a very high bar,* Senior mentions several different feelings you may be experiencing during your fourth trimester. If you feel any of the below, know you are definitely not alone!

1. Anxiety. How am I going to do everything I need to do for this child?
2. Panic. I can't do it all, and I'm freaking out!
3. Anguish. My baby's crying, and I can't get him/her to stop. This is killing me!
4. Confusion. Is it time to feed my baby, or not feed my baby?
5. Stress. There's so much responsibility being a parent, and the pressure is super intense.
6. Marital dissatisfaction. I'm doing the best I can right now, why can't my partner step it up?
7. Uncertainty. I don't know how to be a parent, but apparently everyone else knows how I should be a parent. I just need some room to figure it out myself! Or should I listen to those who know better? And if so, so whom? Everyone has a conflicting opinion on everything.

Add your own to the list:

8. ____

9. ____

10. ____

Welcome back to Acing the Forth Trimester! Let's get back to work.

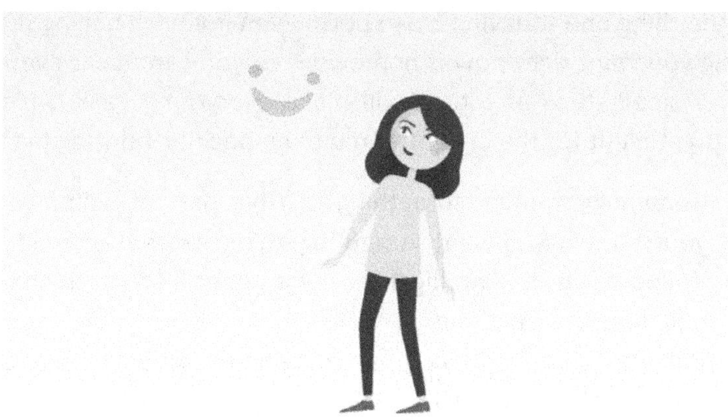

It takes a lot of willpower to do *anything* during the fourth trimester, and willpower functions like a muscle. The more you use it, the stronger it becomes. It also means that we can strengthen it, little by little. In the following clip, Stanford health psychologist Kelly McGonigal speaks about willpower as a bodily process and how we can use this to our advantage. In the exercise that follows, we'll be looking at the power of small steps in helping you pump up your willpower, to shape the forth trimester into what you want it to be.

Watch 'The Willpower Instinct' presented by Kelly McGonigal on YouTube.

11 Ideas to help build your willpower (even with a newborn!)

Here's the thing about having a newborn: Even if you're nailing it, it's a lot of hard work. The last thing you want right now is homework so you can nail it even more. But increasing your willpower small steps at a time will make *everything* easier, from brushing your teeth to getting up at night for the billionth time to go pacifier-hunting in the dark.

1. Genuinely wanting something is a big part of willpower; the more you clarify to yourself *why* you want something, the greater your ability to will it into being.
2. Willpower is like intelligence. It's a general strength that you can build, and it can help improve anything.
3. Willpower can predict how successful someone will be in the future; a better predictor than even IQ!
4. Willpower is about remembering what our goals are and following through on them.
    (Plus: Check out our Achieve Your Goals course   )
5. Willpower is thinking long-term satisfaction, as opposed to short-term instant gratification.
6. When I use willpower in my relationships, I can focus more on my partner and friends and give them the attention they deserve.
7. It makes sense that my willpower muscle gets tired a lot; the society we live in offers non-stop temptations. I need to forgive myself for lapses.
8. Grabbing a nap in the middle of the day does not mean I'm lazy. It means recharging my willpower in order to function healthfully!
    (Plus: Check out our Mindfulness for Beginners course   )

Add some of your ideas:

9. ____

10. ____

11. ____

In a previous session, we outlined what some of our fourth trimester challenges are. But how do you go about actively forming a change? Willpower. It's a muscle you can build to help you make the right choices. Thing is, many postnatal women have a hard time finding the will to find a clean shirt, let alone the energy to begin building muscles. But the truth is, research on developing willpower paints a much more modest picture.

You won't be pumping iron or working up a healthy sweat. **Instead of imagining a Schwarzenegger-esque body builder, you would be more aligned with the science if you envisioned a regular person– such as yourself–walking one lap around the living room each day.**

For example, in her book *The Willpower Instinct,* Stanford health psychologist Kelly McGonigal writes about the power of committing to a small act of self-control, like cutting back on sweets or improving your posture.

These seemingly insignificant tasks may appear unimportant when it comes to the bigger willpower challenges, but it turns out that they do improve your overall inner strength.

As an example, McGonigal presents a study conducted at Northwestern University that tested this notion with two weeks of willpower training to reduce violence against romantic partners.

In the study, a group of participants were asked to change small habits in their day, such as using their non-dominant hand for tasks, or saying "yes" instead of "yeah." After two weeks, this group showed a reduction in physical violence as a response to typical triggering events, in comparison to the control group. Meaning, the simple acts they were asked to execute for two weeks strengthened their overall self-discipline and they were less likely to lose control. Their willpower muscle had become stronger. Imagine what this did to their self-esteem.

Now, we don't usually respond with violence over spilling some milk; but that was before the hormones and the chafing and time it took to pump the milk or to sterilize the bottle. More than ever, the fourth trimester is a time to overcome the kneejerk reaction to react strongly. The simple act of training the self-control muscle, even by committing to a small exercise, gives us more willpower.

Why is that?

When we train our brains to pause and notice what we are about to do, we prevent automatic responses. If I'm hungry, will I grab a king-sized candy bar, or throw together a tuna-melt? Which hand will I use to eat breakfast? Although these tasks can be challenging at times, they are not overwhelming, and are less likely to trigger strong feelings. Little by little, small and mundane tasks will help you increase your willpower. And as that occurs, you'll find that you have increased willpower in other areas, as well.

Shape your fourth trimester so it's not a blur of automatic responses, but rather a series deliberate decisions.

EXERCISE

Right now, perform one set of Kegels, put your phone on silent so you're not constantly refreshing Twitter, or breathe deeply and deliberately. As you're doing that, **take an awesome selfie** to serve as your reminder that by actively exercising self-control in any area, you'll strengthen your overall willpower. Share your selfie with the Buddy and Soul community! Tag us on Instagram and Twitter @Buddy_N_Soul, using the #BuddynSoulExpecting. By sharing with us on social media, not only can you help others with their personal journeys, you can read about those facing similar challenges.

TIPS

Tip 1: Although the idea that a simple task can increase your willpower seems silly, try it — for a week, or longer. It'll pay off.

Tip 2: Keep your willpower exercises gentle and fun so they don't tire you out for your regular responsibilities.

Tip 3: Come back to your journal and update how far you've come with strengthening your willpower muscle.

11 Signs that your willpower is like a muscle

Even though willpower is an abstract skill, it functions very similarly to a physical muscle. Here are a few examples how.

1. When you stop exercising your willpower, it will become flabby and weak.
2. When you push your muscles to their limit, they get stronger. The more you use your willpower, the stronger it will be.
3. If you push your muscles too far, they will be strained and injured. If put on overdrive, willpower can be exhausted and damaged. Sometimes you need to allow yourself to have some fun.
4. Just like eating healthy and exercising are good for your muscles, leading a healthy lifestyle nurtures your brain and gives it the inner strength to utilize willpower effectively.
5. You use your muscles to accomplish many types of tasks. Willpower will help you succeed in all aspects of your life.
6. Sometimes you treat your muscles to a gift – a massage! Give yourself a gift and a pat on the back when you have successfully used willpower to accomplish something.
7. Just like muscles cannot function without ligaments and bones, willpower cannot be employed without self-awareness, patience and perseverance.
8. There are no shortcuts to getting big muscles. It is hard and tiring work! Building up your willpower is tiring and hard as well, but will lead to lasting results.

Add your own:

9. ____

10. ____

11. ____

Can dealing with minor obstacles help new moms deal with the Big Things?

Runners train to prepare themselves for a marathon, and perhaps postpartum moms can take a page out of their book. Afterall, if anything is a solid metaphor for parenting it's that it's a marathon, not a sprint. Can tackling smaller obstacles help you get in shape for when you need a willpower-marathon? Or are you already *in* the marathon, and from here on in it's just about survival?

For:

1. Tackling minor challenges (sitting up straight, doing Kegels, brushing your teeth) will sharpen your problem-solving skills. By the time a huge challenge comes along, you'll have had ample practice dealing with tough situations.
2. Dealing with minor challenges will build your confidence to face the bigger challenges (like standing up to a rude nurse or doctor) head-on.
3. Getting minor obstacles out of the way will give you the time and the energy to focus on the greater challenges of your fourth trimester, like maneuvering your life with a baby in it.

Add your own:

4. ____

Against:

1. Major obstacles are nothing like minor obstacles. When you encounter the real deal, you're not going to know what hit you.
2. Being able to deal with minor obstacles by yourself may prevent you from seeking assistance when a big challenge comes along. After all, willpower is finite and you might need someone else to help you supplement your limited supply.
3. After successfully overcoming temptations or minor obstacles, you develop a false hope that you can easily deal with any challenge that comes your way. When a major obstacle comes along, you will be discouraged when dealing with it isn't as manageable.

Add your own:

4. ____

The surprising thing I did to strengthen my willpower muscle

Thinking of willpower as a muscle is empowering and also opens up a new range of possibilities for how to use and strengthen it. Use your journal to describe what you've found helpful in learning to strengthen your willpower muscle, especially during this trying time of being post-birth.

Direct message us YOUR story @Buddy_N_Soul on Instagram and be anonymously featured for a chance to **win a Buddy&Soul three month free membership.**

STRATEGY 5: Dare to be supported

Getting support is different—and often more encompassing—than getting help.

Have you ever heard the African (and/or Native American) proverb that "it takes a village to raise a child?" When you hear it pre-birth it sounds silly, and when you hear it post birth it sounds ridiculously understated. Who knew raising one child (let alone two or three) would be so much work? It almost makes you wish *you* had a mommy to help you every single moment (without overstepping her bounds or getting on your nerves, that is).

I remember when I was two weeks postpartum and my sister in-law came over for a surprise visit. There I was sitting in my bed at 11:30 in the morning completely topless, covered in milk, and nursing. I had literally been sitting there for the past three hours… nursing. I was dirty, starving, and exhausted. Needless to say, I needed support, and was so glad she had anticipated that; I hadn't known how to ask for it.

We all need help after birth. The first days, weeks, and sometimes months after birth can be tough. That's where physical and emotional support from the outside are a must. In fact, as little as talking to a friend on the phone can help cheer you up and feel positive, according to research from the University of Toronto and Women's College Research Institute. (Dennis & Dowswell, 2013, p. 2).

Some people know to offer help and others tend to shy away because they don't want to 'bother you' too much post-baby, or they don't know what help to offer. Babycenter.com describes the Hispanic tradition of *Cuarentena*, "a period of approximately 40 days (6 weeks) during which the birth mother abstains from sex and is solely dedicated to breastfeeding and taking care of her baby and herself. During this time, other members of the family pitch in to cook, clean, and take care of other children, if there are any."

This lovely tradition bypasses the social pressure to jump back on your feet, and the personal struggle of needing help and not knowing how to ask for it. So go get yourself a little *Cuarentena* from your family and friends when you need it. If entire cultures developed this tradition, it's probably okay to feel a little overwhelmed at the enormity of having a new baby.

Note that support can be defined in many ways, and there's no weakness in asking for any of them. Some women gain support through talking about their feelings. Some women hate talking about their feelings and are looking solely for physical support. Others prefer getting together with other new moms, hearing about others' experiences online, or meeting up with a single friend for coffee, to remind them that they are people, too, and not just nursing machines. The important thing is to draw on all the resources available to you. Some new moms, for example, may have helpful parents living close by, and others may not. Some may have a partner who is gung-ho about diaper changes, while others may be single moms. **Whatever your resources are, it's important to utilize them right now during your time of need and not carry the burden of new-mommy-hood by yourself. You deserve it!**

EXERCISE

Step 1: **Answer the survey question below** in your journal to help you evaluate how you feel toward asking for help.

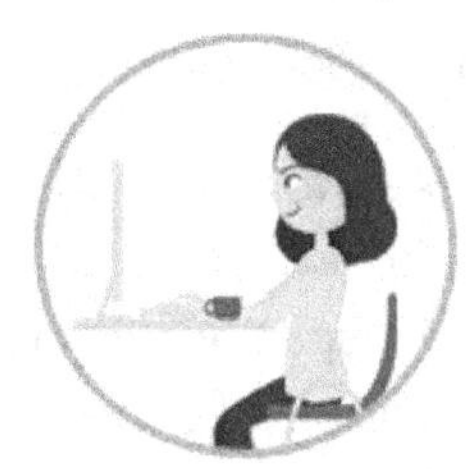

To what extent do these thoughts regarding asking for help describe you?

1. I don't have anyone that can help me
2. I don't trust others; I can do a better job myself
3. I'm really fine, I don't need support
4. I don't want to be a burden on anyone
5. I don't like feeling beholden to someone
6. I ask for help, no problem

Step 2: Reflecting back on your answers to the survey, **how are your thoughts and feelings toward asking for help helping or hindering you?** Also, are they 100% true? Can you think of a possible exception to what you ranked the highest? One person who *can* help you, or to whom you *wouldn't* feel beholden? Record your answers in your journal.

TIPS

Tip 1: If you have a hard time asking for help, designate one person, such as your partner or a friend, to be the asker for you.

Tip 2: Imagine a friend was asking you for help postnatal, what would your response be?

6 Practical ways to get help as a new mama

Every new mama needs help after birth. Rather than crossing your fingers and hoping that help will knock at the door, here are some helpful tips for getting the help you need.

1. Ask for help. Although this may seem a silly first tip, without it, nothing else can follow. If you do not ask for help, there is no guarantee that help will come.
2. Be specific with your needs. Rather than give a general call for help, be detailed: Do you need a meal, or someone to wash your dishes, or just company?
3. Delegate. Know your resources and how to best use them. One friend may really enjoy holding babies, while another friend may be a master chef. Delegate appropriate tasks to friends that will enjoy doing them. This also has the added benefit of not getting 5 meals on one day, and then no meals for the rest of the week.

Can you think of any others?

4. ____

5. ____

6. ____

Is there any point in asking my family for help with the baby?

We all hate that feeling that comes from asking for help and being rejected. If our families have let us down in the past, why would we want to make ourselves vulnerable to that again? And yet, who knows – maybe with a new baby on the scene, things will be different.

For:

1. Most people, including my family, are totally oblivious to my actual needs, but they genuinely want to help. I'll share what I need and see what happens.
2. If I never ask, there's zero chance I'll get help. If I do ask, at least there's a chance.
3. As long as you carefully consider who to ask for what type of help, you may be surprised. A totally unhelpful mom can suddenly become a doting grandmother.
4. Sure, but don't ask everyone for all types of help. Your mother in law may be the right person to babysit, while your own mother can help with grocery shopping (and nothing else). Play to their strengths, making them work for you.

Add your own idea:

5. ____

Against:

1. People with normative families can't imagine the toxicity of some people. Asking for help is just inviting that into your life. I'd rather be overwhelmed than poisoned.
2. I have enough feelings on my plate. Do I really want to add rejection—from those who are supposed to be closest to me—as well?
3. Even if they would come through, ugh, who wants family around? I have enough drama from my toddler trying to adjust to a newborn. Don't need to manufacture more drama than that, for some slight help that will likely come at a cost.

Add your own idea:

7. ____

How I overcame my shyness to ask for help

Asking for help can be hard, and having a baby can be hard, and being shy can be hard. Combining all three can seem impossible to overcome! So if you've done it, write in your journal about how, and help inspire others who feel too shy to ask for help!

Direct message us YOUR story @Buddy_N_Soul on Instagram and be anonymously featured for a chance to **win a Buddy&Soul three month free membership.**

How my outgoing nature let me ask for help

Unapologetically outgoing women can be called rude, stuck-up, sometimes even Captain Marvel... But one thing they always have going for them is that they know how to ask for what they need. Write in your journal about how your own outgoing nature helped you ask for help after giving birth, and maybe help inspire others to embrace their Marvelous, outgoing selves.

Direct message us YOUR story @Buddy_N_Soul on Instagram and be anonymously featured for a chance to **win a Buddy&Soul three month free membership.**

DRIVING THE MESSAGE HOME

A big part of getting the support you really need is asking for help. Family and friends are not mind readers and cannot intuit what it is you need.   They could guess of course, or they could pass, assuming that if you needed the help you would ask for it. According to Amanda Palmer, American singer-songwriter, there is an art when it comes to asking for help, and an art when help is given to you.

Watch 'The Art of Asking' presented by Amanda Palmer on YouTube.

In today's day and age, asking is considered a shameful thing. Begging should be avoided at all cost. And yet, is asking for something really a shameful thing? According to Palmer, who led the first people-sponsored-label project, where her fans donated over a million dollars, asking is a way to connect to others in a very deep way. The very act of asking means making ourselves vulnerable to another. And it is through this deep vulnerability that connection is forged. Even those who have little to give will give gladly when they are asked. They want to have the connection. So take a lesson from Palmer, and ask for help. Let your family and friends know how they can best help you during this postnatal period and beyond. Allow yourself to become vulnerable and make truly deep connections. Don't wait for the help to come on its own.

Should new moms ask for help and risk rejection? Is that art?

In Amanda Palmer's TED Talk, *The Art of Asking*, she emphasizes the incredible art that comes from asking for help and receiving help. In her opinion, asking is not shameful, it's an expression of connection. But do new moms need this added pressure of asking? What if they're rejected? It's hard enough to face that when you're *not* pumped up on hormones and an erratic sleep schedule (at best).

For:

1. Asking involves creative expression.
2. All art involves vulnerability and the possibility of rejection.
3. This is the ability to create connection, even with total strangers. Now that is art!

Add your own:

4. ____

Against:

1. Asking is an art? Then it's the modern kind that uses trash and dirty diapers.
2. There's nothing beautiful about asking. People who love me should offer to help.
3. Asking for help feels terrible and involves rejection. Maybe that's part of being an artist, but it's also why I never became a painter.

Add your own:

4. ____

Should you continue practicing Acing the Fourth Trimester?

You are totally busy with your new baby, and in the rare moments *they're* asleep and you're *not*, you prefer to Netflix and Chill. But here are some reasons why it may be worth it to check in with Acing the Fourth Trimester, instead. Or, in addition to; you're a mom, you multitask now.

For:

1. It will help me embrace the unknowns of motherhood.
2. It will help me make sense of my feelings.
3. It provides helpful tools to all new moms, even if this isn't their first baby.
4. It can help me drop my negative feelings and help me replace them with more positive.

Add your own opinion:

5. ____

Against:

1. Off the bat the course tells me I can't be a perfect mom. It's kinda disheartening.
2. I don't have time to practice it – my baby demands my time all day, and what's left of my day is dedicated to alone-bathroom-time.
3. I'm a mom – that means I know innately what I need in order to be a good mom, I don't need a course!
4. I'm so used to being imperfect – I stink at everything I do. Who needs this course to drive it home?

Add your own opinion:

5. ____

My first-born was what we'd call an easy baby. She slept well, ate every three hours, and was overall content. I thought I was the most talented mother until my second came along. She didn't sleep well, ate ravenously all the time, and was fussy. Only then did I realize that when it comes to parenting there are two people in the relationship; and therefore, I have control over my side of the partnership, and zero control over the other side.

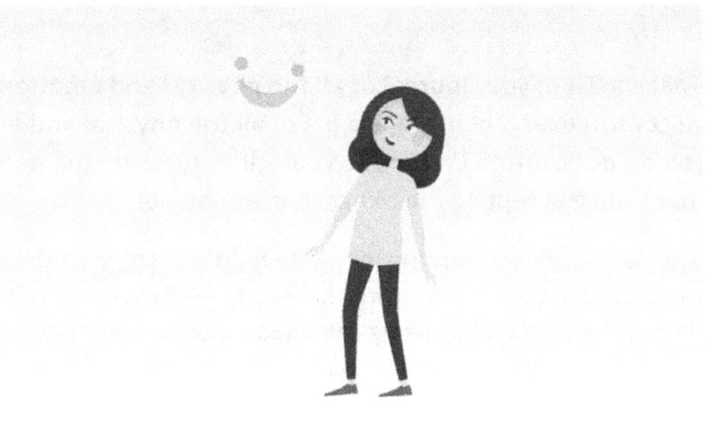

Being a parent means embracing what you have control over, and letting go of what you don't. This is true for physical things, and for emotional things as well. For example, a new mom can decide what she wants to wear, whether or not she wants to nurse, if she remains calm or becomes enraged, and if she will smile or scowl at her baby. She cannot decide however, how long her baby will sleep, if her baby will agree to her eating schedule, and if her baby is gassy, colicky, downright grumpy, or as smiley as a cartoon newborn.

According to *Present Perfect: A Mindfulness Approach to Letting Go of Perfectionism and the Need for Control* by self-help author Pavel Somov Ph.D., licensed psychologist and mindfulness expert, you have two choices when faced with something uncontrollable: "You can try to control it, which is an anxiety-fraught delusion. Or you can try to control your reaction to the uncontrollable, which can be acceptance, courage, and possibly a sense of fun" (Somov, p. 158). **Therefore, it's time to let go of what we cannot control and embrace what we can.** Not only will it reduce stress, but also it can allow us to make changes in the areas that we can control, ourselves.

For me, that meant realizing that it wasn't that I forgot how to be a good, effective mother, it's just that there was a different person in the relationship with me this time around. And while I couldn't control how fussy she was, I could certainly put *myself* in a brief time-out, to regain my composure before dealing with her.

EXERCISE

Step 1: **Make a list in your journal of all the physical and emotional things that you have control over. Then, make a list of all the physical and emotional things you do not control.** Commit to yourself to focus on the items you do have control over while accepting the things that you do not.

Step 2: Look up a funny parenting meme to help you laugh at those things you can't control! Share your meme with the Buddy and Soul community! Tag us on Instagram and Twitter @Buddy_N_Soul, using the #BuddynSoulExpecting. By sharing with us on social media, not only can you help others with their personal journeys, you can read about those facing similar challenges.

My personal favorite? "My kids are the reason I wake up every morning. Really freakin' early… Every. Single. Morning."

TIPS

Tip 1: Laughter is a great way to manage those things you can't control.

Tip 2: Smile through it. You'll feel a lot happier.

7 Ways for new moms to release control

Having a baby is so momentous, that any bit of control we can garner is seized with two hands. Except… that doesn't happen very often, considering you can't control when the baby will come, what the experience will be like, when you'll get to go home, how she'll eat, sleep, or play, or whether you'll ever sleep again, at all. Having so little control over your life can be difficult in and of itself, and here are some ways to help ease that feeling of spinning out.

1. Open your mind to other alternatives beyond your own. Yes, there are other opinions and schools of thought out there when it comes to parenting. Once there are other possibilities, being in control of one specifically desired outcome feels less necessary.
2. Think of yourself as plotting a course, rather than wandering aimlessly. There is a logic to your child, you just haven't figured it out quite yet. It might take years to map out just the broad strokes, but you're in it for the long run, right?
3. Be mindful of the moment. In this particular moment, there are things you can and cannot control. So even if you can't control how long it takes the baby to nurse, you *can* control how frustrated you get and what you're going to do while he's at it (pro tip: you're not required to lovingly stare at him as he suckles from your bosom—or bottle. You can watch TV, go online, or read a book to your older kids).
4. Squeeze your hands really tight together into fists, and then release. You feel that physical sense of release? Well, you can create emotional release by focusing your mind on all the overwhelming aspects of life right now, and letting go of emotional control.

Do you have any other suggestions?

5. ____

6. ____

7. ____

Can new moms control their baby by controlling the environment?

Everyone knows you can't control what kid you get, and no amount of shouting will actually help you effectively control your kid. But what about if you doctor the environment, so as to limit their range of choice? Would that work, and how early can you start?

For:

1. I am in control of me, who is in control of my baby's environment, which in turn controls of my baby. A darkened room will ensure a longer naptime.
2. The baby is helpless without me. Not to be cynical, but what's that if not control?
3. I can decide when he's in bed, when he nurses, and how much. That sounds like control.

Add your own:

4. ____

Against:

1. Baby's don't only respond to environment. You can darken a room all you want, but that baby will keep on screaming.
2. I can try my best to control the environment, but never completely! How can I possibly control whether or not he catches a cold, gets gassy, or is legitimately hungry every 30 minutes?
3. I can control when the baby's in bed, but I can't control whether or not she sleeps, or how much she cries. That's exactly where I need to relinquish control.

Add your own:

4. ____

I released control... But nothing changed!

So you took a deep breath, said here-goes-nothing, and... There went nothing, because everything stayed the same? Write about your experience (and maybe even frustration!) in your journal. Maybe this can help you see what's holding you back.

By loading kids with high expectations and micromanaging their lives at every turn, parents aren't actually helping. At least, that's how Julie Lythcott-Haims sees it. With passion and wry humor, the former Dean of Freshmen at Stanford makes the case for parents to stop defining their children's success via grades and test scores, or how well they sleep and how early they smile. Instead, she says, they should focus on providing the oldest idea of all: unconditional love.

And the basis of unconditional love? Acceptance of who our child is; this involves letting go of trying to control our children, and letting them evolve into their own unique self. Even an infant exercises her need to be in control; they know innately when they need to eat, sleep, or poop. So let's try to take control of what we can: ourselves.

Watch 'How to Raise Successful Kids- Without Over-Parenting' presented by Julie Lythcott-Haims on YouTube.

Lythcott-Haims is wrong; we need to control our children!

In Julie Lythcott-Haims' TED Talk, *How to raise successful kids without over parenting*, Lythcott-Haims emphasizes the need to allow our kids to be themselves and for parents not to hover over them all the time. How does that fit with your own parenting philosophy?

For:

1. Babies especially need us to control them; otherwise how else will they learn?
2. Forget about babies, I want my adult kids to obey everything I say!
3. Obedience is way better than the freedom to choose; how can a kid choose correctly anyway?
4. I don't like all this fluff. If I'm not in control my kid will be in control, and for a seven-year-old, that means chaos. Let alone a newborn.

Add your own idea:

5. ____

Against:

1. I shudder at the very word 'control.' I won't let them play with forks and electricity sockets, but why should I dictate their likes and dislikes?
2. My parents tried controlling me and I hated it, and rebelled *hard*. Why would I do that to my own child?
3. Self-efficacy comes from learning how to do things on one's own. I'm way into that.
4. It may challenge my own control issues, but I like this whole philosophy; let our kids be who they want to be, not who I try to make them be.

Add your own idea:

5. ____

STRATEGY 7: Establish some healthy eating habits

We know! That title… But don't nope-out quite yet; just hear us out.

With all the constant nursing and/or bottle feeding, you are doing your best to nurture your little baby around the clock. When it comes to nurturing yourself, however, it can become a lot harder. You're like the main character in a 90s action film. You're on a countdown timer between feedings and diaper changes and other responsibilities, so when that little voice tells you to cut a nice salad and make each bite a mindful experience, all you can do is dramatically declare into your earpiece, *"there's no time!"* and grab something that can be microwaved in under 2 minutes and consumed as you're falling asleep. And if you do have the luxury of a meal? You're not exactly tempted to waste it on chia seed butter on whole Ezekiel bread. And you know what? We're so with you.

But, we also know that now is the time to focus on your wellbeing, and to **establish healthy habits that can positively impact the postnatal experience**.

The last thing you probably want to worry about right now is your own wellbeing, especially when it comes to something like healthy eating habits. But a big change, such as giving birth, is one of the most effective times to establish a new habit. **And although it may take an extreme amount of effort on your part, focusing on health can make a big impact on you and your baby (who directly benefits from your wellbeing).**

Several major studies, from universities and institutes all around the world, have dedicated their research to the benefits of proper nutrition in women during the postnatal period. The science says that good nutrition can have a positive impact on your mood. This is a helpful tidbit to keep in mind at all times, but especially now that your body is craving nutrients and your emotional state may be a little rocky. What, when, and how frequently you eat can all contribute to your overall sense of well-being. For some women, the challenge is to curb the constant urge for sugar and comfort foods; for others, it's remembering to eat when your days and nights just feel like a big timeless blur. But over-eating, under-eating, and eating poor-quality foods can all wreak havoc on your emotional state: low levels of omega-3, lack of vitamin D and other trace minerals, and high amounts of dietary added sugars are all associated with increased odds of postpartum depression (Markhus et al., 2013), (Ellsworth-Bower & Corwin, 2012), (Gangwisch et al., 2015),

This does not mean suddenly eating only home-cooked, macrobiotic foods. You did just have a baby! But you can take some small steps toward creating better habits that will stick with you even past the fourth trimester.

EXERCISE

Make a list in your journal of at least 3 small, healthy, eating habits you'd like to establish for yourself. This can range from, *'an apple a day,'* to *'drink lots of water'* to *'I will not skip breakfast!'* Then **choose one to begin implementing today**! Share your inspiring picture with the Buddy and Soul community! Tag us on Instagram and Twitter @Buddy_N_Soul, using the #BuddynSoulExpecting. By sharing with us on social media, not only can you help others with their personal journeys, you can read about those facing similar challenges.

TIPS

Tip 1: For more on habits, be sure to check out our Habit Workshop course. 

Tip 2: Use your calendar feature on your phone to send yourself reminders to keep up with your habit!

What's holding you back from healthy eating habits?

With all the publicity nowadays for staying fit and eating nutritiously, we've probably all been exposed to these messages. And yet, it can be so hard to change the way we eat! What are some of the obstacles that hold you back from developing healthier eating habits?

1. My intense craving for sugar and caffeine … especially now. When you're nursing, a banana just doesn't cut it.
2. I'm already on the (insert name of diet here), what else can I do?
3. I don't believe I can do it.
4. Low motivation. I just had a baby! All I care about is sleep.
5. Nutrition is not as important as everyone makes it out to be.

What else is holding you back?

6. ____

7. ____

8. ____

7 Ways for new moms to implement healthy eating habits

It's so easy to set healthy eating habits… and we'll do that just as soon as we get a good night's sleep. Well, unfortunately there's no guarantee as to when that's gonna kick in, so we've gathered a few easy tips that will allow you to begin implementing healthy eating habits today.

1. Make your habit goals **SMART**: Specific, Measurable, Agreed upon, Realistic, Time-bound. Meaning, don't decide *today I'll eat good*; decide instead, *when I wake up, I will have just one pop-tart and then an apple.*
2. Start with tiny steps; if the step is tiny (like filling a water bottle), you'll have a lot less resistance from procrastination.
3. Get a buddy. Having a partner on board with you for eating healthily together can help you stay motivated and implement healthy eating habits.
4. Choose an obvious cue/trigger. For example, drinking a glass of water every time you finish nursing or feeding your baby will help you stay hydrated, and gives you an easy way to follow through.

Can you think of any others?

5. ____

6. ____

7. ____

How my days changed because of one new habit

Days and nights are practically interchangeable these days, but what's the one new habit that helped you find some light in the endless night, some order in the chaos that is life with a newborn? Write about it in your journal!

Direct message us YOUR story @Buddy_N_Soul on Instagram and be anonymously featured for a chance to **win a Buddy&Soul three month free membership.**

It's amazing how from the tiniest beginnings we can create significant changes. In this inspirational and informative TED Talk, BJ Fogg explains how behavior changes, such as flossing, or eating healthy are not complicated, they're simply systematic. And his simple solution for creating new habits? Tiny steps. Because they do not intimidate you they are easy to set and maintain. From one pushup a day to 65, Fogg takes us on a journey through building a successful routine through habit formation that ultimately creates big changes; the perfect backdrop for becoming a more nutrition-and-health conscious you.

Watch 'Forget Big Changes, Start with a Tiny Habit' presented by BJ Fogg at TEDxFremont on YouTube.

I took my first nutrition-step thanks to Fogg

Did Fogg help inspire you to make a nutrition-change, during what is one of the most hectic times of your life? Write about this experience in your journal!

I took my first nutrition-step thanks to Fogg

Did Fogg help inspire you to make a nutrition-change, during what is one of the most hectic times of your life? Write about this experience in your journal!

STRATEGY 8: Call out your false beliefs

We all hold certain assumptions and beliefs about ourselves and the world around us. Often these are both negative and false. And yet, we still operate upon them. Some apt examples might be:

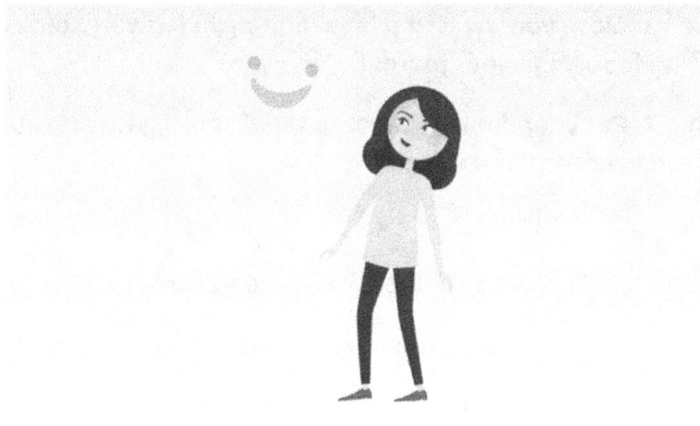

- "I'm the worst; I just wait for my baby to fall asleep so I can be myself again."
- "I'm so fat, and I'm not even pregnant to justify it."
- "I just ate a whole bag of chips. I'm disgusting."
- "I'm a terrible mom, I can't even nurse my baby."

Some of these come from our own perceptions and life experiences or from internalizing messages that others (parents, teachers, "friends," ex-partners, etc.) have sent us. These disempowering mantras block us from making progress and enjoying this period after birth. They suck up a lot of mental energy that would be better spent elsewhere.

Just like we declutter our wardrobe, weeding out garments which no longer fit or no longer serve us, it's time to declutter and re-examine the premises and assumptions we have about our parenthood. Keep the ones that are good for you and get rid of the rest. It's a shame to walk around with the weight of false beliefs. It's a weight you should never have to carry, and it's often heavy enough to squash any hope of finding peace.

If you think you don't love your baby as much as you "should," you are undermining your ability to function as a mother. And if you're nursing despite the fact that it makes you hate yourself and your baby, because you have this notion that that's what so-called good moms do, you might be dying on a hill for something you don't really believe in.

In the words of self-development author Brian Tracy, "if you believe yourself to be limited in some way, whether or not it is true, it becomes true for you" (*Goals!*, p. 42).

So let's get started on getting rid of those negative thoughts and mantras.

A helpful framework for questioning beliefs comes from leading author and self-inquiry teacher Byron Katie. In her method of self-inquiry which she calls "The Work," Katie puts forth four crucial questions which you can ask yourself about any belief you're holding:

1. Is it true?

2. Can you absolutely know that it's true?

3. How do you react, what happens, when you believe that thought?

4. Who would you be without the thought?

A word of warning: decluttering your false beliefs may be harder than you think, but not too hard for us to suggest it. It requires acknowledging that your beliefs may not be true and coming to terms with the price you've already paid for holding this faith. It does pay off, I promise.

EXERCISE

Step 1: **Close your eyes and let a limiting belief you hold come to the surface. Write it down in your journal.**

Step 2: **Put your limiting belief to the test** using Byron Katie's 4 prompts. Write down your response to each:

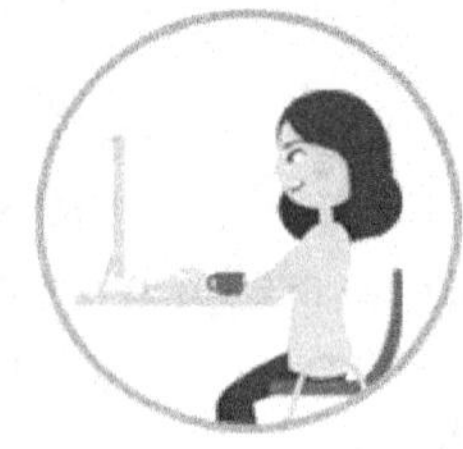

1. Is it true?

2. Can you absolutely know that it's true?

3. How do you react, what happens, when you believe that thought?

4. Who would you be without the thought?

TIPS

Tip 1: Ridding yourself of false beliefs doesn't happen overnight. Be forgiving, but persistent.

Tip 2: You might be feeling overwhelmed by the price you already paid when you followed this false belief. Let bygones be bygones. You cannot change the past, but you can minimize this price going forward and make sure not to make the same mistake twice.

Tip 3: Another way to get rid of assumptions and false beliefs is by reframing them. Instead of "I'm a shapeless blob," you could view yourself more favorably: "I don't have the body I did at senior prom, but this baby is worth a few years of fighting to get back in shape." Check out our Everyday Reframing course 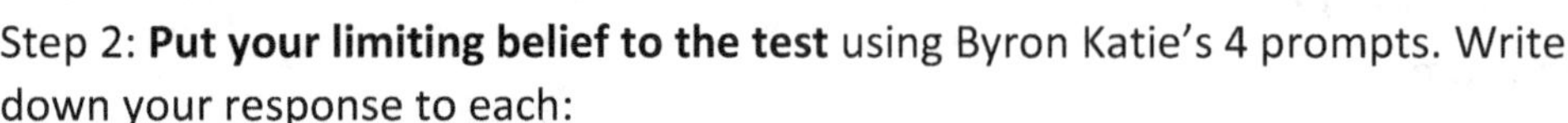 for more.

6 Tips for disorganized moms to declutter false beliefs

False beliefs can strike anyone, regardless of organization level. But here are a few tricks for the particularly disorganized moms among us—whether new or seasoned—to declutter false beliefs that are keeping us back.

1. Don't believe everything you hear (or read). Anyone can write a blog, post an opinion piece, or loudly cry on a Facebook group that anyone who does sleep training is a bad mom. Doesn't make it true.
2. Empirical data is, well, empirical, but not everyone is suited to pouring over verbose texts just to determine whether good mothers let their babies cry it out. Listening to friends with experience is a great way to challenge your beliefs in an easy, contained way.
3. Hide reminder notes to yourself about the belief you want to change. 'Good mothers get a day off!' or 'crying≠trauma' can go a long way when you find it in a forgotten, unexpected place.

Do you have any tips?

4. ____

5. ____

6. ____

What are your greatest barriers at decluttering false beliefs?

Everyone has them, but somehow, that doesn't help with dealing with them, or getting rid of them. What are some of the things that hold you back from decluttering false beliefs?

1. But… I can't get rid of that pestering 'but' thought that follows any positive thought I have about myself.
2. The belief is reinforced by my environment. Maybe it's not so false after all if *everyone* things I'm momming all wrong?
3. It would require too many changes to challenge the belief.
4. I don't have the money to challenge my beliefs.

Add your own:

5. ____

6. ____

7. ____

When I finally confronted my false belief, and defeated it

Regardless of how big it is, confronting a false belief is incredibly hard. It requires you to look deeply and honestly into yourself and change something fundamental about how you think. What was your false belief, and how did you defeat it? Write your story in your journal!

DRIVING THE MESSAGE HOME

Sometimes we don't even realize all the false messages we are storing and how they are impacting our daily lives. Neuroanatomist Jill Bolte Taylor knew intellectually how impactful false beliefs were, but it wasn't until she had a stroke that she was able to understand experientially what life looks like without any previous memories or messages. She describes in amusing detail the morning of the stroke and the freedom of "losing 37 years of emotional baggage". Can you imagine, even momentarily what your life would look like if you could lose a lifetime of your own false beliefs and emotional baggage?

Watch 'My Stroke of Insight' presented by Jill Bolte Taylor on YouTube.

Can low mental energy really affect my parenting?

There are plenty of highly successful people out there with a lot on their minds, little sleep, and newborns. I'm a multitasker, my mom is a multitasker and so is my best friend- why do I need to up my mental energy if I'm doing well enough, all things considered?

For:

1. Are you sure what you have now is success?
2. If you think you're succeeding now, just imagine what it could be like if your mind was clear!
3. You've got nothing to lose. If you declutter you may surprise yourself.

Add your own thoughts:

4. ____

Against:

1. My spouse and my boss (and most everyone around me) can do a gazillion things at once, so there's no reason I shouldn't be able to.
2. Just because I'm thinking of things from the past, doesn't mean I won't be successful. If I'm good at what I do, what does it matter what's going on inside my mind?
3. I don't have the time to try to fool around with changing my mind and my way of thought. I am where I am, there's no way to change it.

Add your own thoughts:

4. ____

STRATEGY 9: Embrace my imperfections

The first few months after birth, it can feel like life has set up cruel, carnivalesque funhouse mirrors of imperfections all around us.

You look one way, and all you can see is how enormous you still are; so you turn to the left, but that way is a reflection of you holding a baby who *won't stop crying no matter what you do*. To the right isn't much better—there it looks like your baby's not gaining enough weight, and regardless of which way you turn, you can't seem to find an aspect of parenting that's going just right.

But a little ironically, an important piece of developing good mothering skills is letting go of the 'perfect' complex. It is impossible when working with children (or anyone for that matter) to get it 100% right 100% of the time. You won't always know when they're hungry, or catch their tired cues before they go ballistic on you, or be able to intuit what's wrong. One of the biggest lies of parenthood is that "a mom always knows." A big part of the time mom is winging it. Sometimes dad will know, and sometimes it will remain a mystery. The best you can do is do the best you can do for them.

And all this is more than just okay, it's the way things should be. All that matters is that you are good enough. That's literally the official term for a healthy, functioning mom: Good enough. Donald Winnicott, an English psychoanalyst who revolutionized the field of parenting-psychology, coined the phrase 'a good enough mother,' to emphasize this exact point: You can't be a perfect parent. Even if you try, you'll fail. And that's fine, because a perfect parent isn't what kids *need*. What they need is a mother who is, simply, good enough. One who loves them enough, feeds them enough, cares for them enough. And that's the type of mother you can be. One of the best lessons you can model for your child is the valuable truth that nobody is perfect, but we love them just the same! It's time to let go of all the guilt that comes with feeling imperfect and embrace the ambiguity of motherhood.

EXERCISE

Imagine you are confiding with a very dear friend some of your imperfections. **Write your imperfections in your journal as you would share them**.

Then, take a moment and think, how would she respond? Would she say, *you're right, you are fat, ugly, a bad mom, and you should probably put your kid up for adoption*. Or would she say, *'honey, you are beautiful, you just had a baby. It will take time to feel like you did before the pregnancy, but your baby is happy and healthy. That's what a good mom does!*

Write her responses to you in your journal.

Then, make a pledge to start thinking about yourself as your loving friend does!

TIPS

Tip 1: Don't choose a judgmental friend! Choose a caring and loving friend who does not judge!

Tip 2: Be as concrete/specific as possible, this way you address your concerns head on.

Tip 3: Remember, a perfect mother does not exist. Good enough is good enough!

I'm a perfectionist I won't aim for "good enough".

The whole concept of 'good enough' seems outrageous to the perfectionist type. Why settle for good enough or even great when you can aim for perfect? After all, it's better to fall a bit short from perfect, than to fall short from good enough, and essentially fail.

For:

1. Seriously, why settle for good enough when you can aim for perfect?
2. Why can't there be such a thing as a perfect parent?
3. If I've become perfect as a partner, and that took work, why can't I be a perfect mom? Babies are much easier!
4. Good enough is an excuse not to try so hard; I want to be a parent who really tries.

What do you think? Add your own:

5. ____

Against:

1. Perfectionism is an excuse to stop trying because it's a goal I can never reach. Good enough, however, is an attainable goal and will keep me striving.
2. Nobody's perfect. If you try, you're only setting yourself up for failure.
3. Better to aim at good enough and likely succeed as opposed to aiming at perfect and surely failing.
4. By definition, the need for perfection is a flaw that will translate into your parenting (like comparing your child to others who are more advanced in certain areas). See? You've already failed.

What do you think? Add your own:

5. ____

10 Signs of a good-enough mom

With all the attachment-focused parenting craze, it's easy to lose perspective of what a realistic parent looks like. A realistic parent is a good-enough parent, and definitely not a perfect parent. Those don't exist in the real world.

1. She takes time for herself.
2. She smiles at her baby.
3. She is attentive to her baby's cries, but isn't a slave to them.
4. She has perspective on what's important (feeding her baby) and what's not (what her mother-in-law thinks about feeding her baby).
5. She asks for help when she needs it.
6. She makes mistakes.
7. She cuts herself some slack.

What makes you a good enough mom?

8. ____

9. ____

10. ____

How I was able to let go of my imperfections

The title is only a few words, but the secret it holds can fill several novels: the journey of letting go of imperfections can take many forms, and each one is a world of success in its own right. Write in your journal about your successful tale of letting go of imperfections and embracing the good-enough life.

Direct message us YOUR story @Buddy_N_Soul on Instagram and be anonymously featured for a chance to **win a Buddy&Soul three month free membership.**

Feelings of imperfection may be surfacing as you tread through this new period in your life. Imperfection of your body, of how you act and respond, even how you feel. And along with imperfection, usually comes feelings of shame and unworthiness. This TED Talk by shame and vulnerability researcher and best-selling author Brené Brown, viewed over three million times, is revolutionary when it comes to embracing shame. It teaches the necessary tools to embrace our shame and imperfection head on. By identifying shame for what it is we are then able to release it. By ignoring shame, it will continue to influence our lives, our choices, and of course our changes. So, take the opportunity to embrace your shame and imperfection; from this place can come courage, compassion, and change.

Watch 'Listening to Shame' presented by Brené Brown on YouTube.

My biggest shame—and how I came to accept it

Shame is a learned construct. Don't get us wrong—it often serves a good and noble purpose (self-cut bangs, I'm looking at you)—but it's not something that is inherently bad. Use your journal to write about how you managed to accept your shame, and acknowledge that while it may not be the best part of you, it's something that you can come to accept.

Direct message us YOUR story @Buddy_N_Soul on Instagram and be anonymously featured for a chance to **win a Buddy&Soul three month free membership.**

STRATEGY 10: (Re-)Shift into the 'mom role'

Before you had the baby, you were a whole person. A daughter, a sister, a friend, a student, a professional, a fan; maybe you were even a mother, but not to this particular kid. And now? You've got another huge role to integrate into your personality. Even if you've done this before with older kids, it's still a big deal. And if it's your first time? It can be overwhelming.

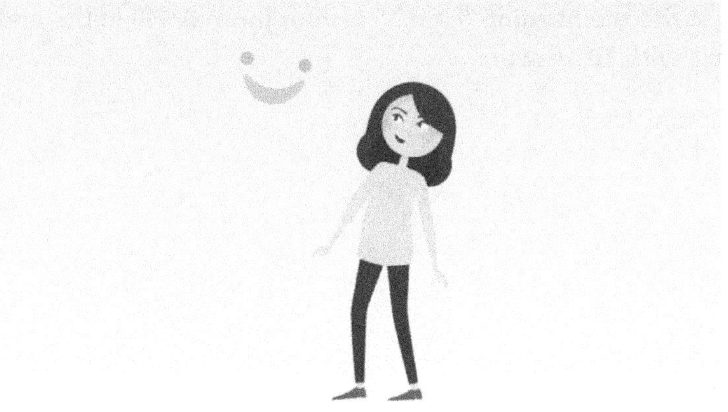

According to The Oxford Handbook of Identity Development, "Identity… is not a static entity, remaining fixed once initial resolutions are made. **Changing life circumstances, coupled with changing biological and psychological needs, will likely spur ongoing identity developments over the course of adulthood years**" (McLean & Syed, 2014, p. 65). As we continue to grow and develop through life, our identity is constantly evolving, like moving from a not-mom to a mom, or a mother of one to a mother of two, etc.

There is a crucial identity shift when becoming a parent, because we suddenly no longer have the luxury to think only for ourselves. We have an additional person (or persons) we are responsible for and must take care of; we now take on, so to speak, a mother's role. This transition can sometimes be a smooth one, and other times, not so much.

It is a big challenge to not only adopt a new identity but also to balance it with your former self: some women are on the career warpath, and as soon as they have their baby all they want is to be a stay-at-home mom. Others (like yours truly), enjoy the blissfulness of being at home with a baby for about six months, and then just *itch* to get back to hanging out with adults who rarely spit up on them. Others find that work and homelife balance perfectly, but need to find a way back to their dance classes in order to feel like themselves again. There are so many parts to your identity, it's only natural that you'll find it challenging to make all the pieces fit neatly again.

Taking the time to process your huge role change is a great way to consciously embrace the ongoing identity struggle you are facing. Identify who you were, what you are now and who you hope to become. Think about how your new identity of being a mom can fit into this picture.

EXERCISE

Step 1: **Write the heading "I am..." in your journal. Fill in the end of the sentence with 10 answers.**

For example: I am...

an exec

a mom

tall

loving

exhausted

Don't stop until you've gotten all the way through.

Step 2: **Then select seven entries with which you least identify and cross them off leaving only the three that you most identified with.**

Step 3: Label the three that are left from 1-3, 1 being the one you identify the most.

Creating this list will help you discern which parts of yourself you most identify with and help bring light to some of the struggles you may undergo when you add 'I am a mom' to it.

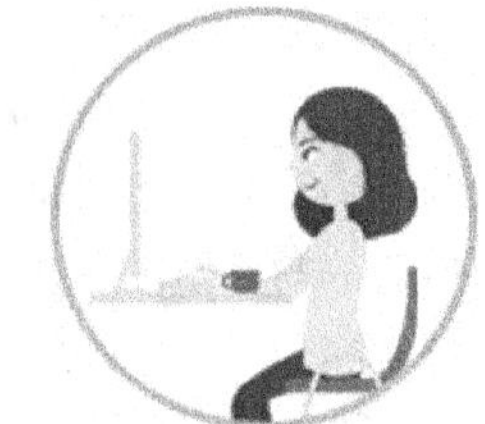

TIPS

Tip 1: Were you surprised at what you identified with most? For more on authenticity and discovering who you are, be sure to take our Cultivating authenticity course.

Tip 2: Don't feel pressured to put "mom" first, or even in your top-3. Some women feel that way, some don't. Both are totally normal and natural.

Tip 3: Remind yourself daily who you really are; this can help you raise your spirits and live a focused day.

7 Reasons you may hate your new 'mom' role

Having a baby and being a mom is exciting, but it's also intimidating and scary. Here are some reasons why being placed in the 'mom' role may not bring up good feelings.

1. Being a mom somehow suddenly comes with a lot of unwanted social pressure. Mommy and Me? Baby and I? Princess and Mama? Newborn Pilates? Gotta catch 'em all.
2. Yes, I'm a mom. I'm also a career woman, partner, and friend. Why does this one suddenly get everyone's focus?
3. The title 'mom' reminds me of my own mother, and I definitely am not ready to give up everything I have going on to be *her*!
4. The word mom is so… permanent. It's so scary thinking that I will bear my tag my whole life.

Add your own:

5. ____

6. ____

7. ____

How much do the following 'roles' define you?

From childhood we've developed many roles that have come to define who we are and how we see ourselves. Now, you've developed a new role: a mom. How much do the following roles define how you see yourself today?

1. The mom role.
2. The spouse/partner role.
3. The professional role.
4. My role as a person, and everything that entails. I don't like this idea of prepackaged roles.

Are there any roles we are missing?

5. ____

6. ____

7. ____

When I realized that I wasn't primarily a mom

Being a mom can be overwhelming (and it can *not* be overwhelming, too; no judgement here), but there usually comes a time in the fourth trimester when you realize you're more than just a mom, and you "snap." You go out and do something to prove to yourself and your surrounding that you're more than just the mother of this beautiful, perfect little creature. What was your moment? What made you re-realize you were more than a mom? Write about this experience in your journal!

Direct message us YOUR story @Buddy_N_Soul on Instagram and be anonymously featured for a chance to **win a Buddy&Soul three month free membership.**

DRIVING THE MESSAGE HOME

We are incredibly impressionable from a young age. From birth we absorb societal expectations and values, taking in what we see around us. These early stigmas and beliefs are ones we are now faced with post-baby. What does it mean to be a mother? Who am I now that I have a child? How do I redefine myself with this new role? These impressionable beliefs we had as children are challenging us today.

Watch 'The Danger of a Single Story' presented by Chimamanda Ngozi Adichie on YouTube.

In this TED Talk, Chimamanda Ngozi Adichie, a black Nigerian novelist, describes writing stories as a child about white, blue eyed children; this is what she read, and this is what she thought life was about. The danger of one narrative, the story we've told ourselves since we were children, is that there is no flexibility. It is incredibly limiting. We expect that things will be the way we experienced life as children, and that is rarely true.

We each have a unique story; several unique stories. How can we let someone else define who we are? Now is the time to become empowered and determine as an adult what you want your narrative to be. Becoming a new mother is about recreating your own story. Deciding how you want it to be, as opposed to what society tells you that you should be.

I realized a troubled narrative thanks to Ngozi Adichie

The problem with our narratives is that they're so much a part of us, we don't ever stop to consider whether they're good, or appropriate, or even true. We just get so used to telling a particular story, it feels true, even when it's not. That's why it's so important to take a few moments and try to realize whether our narrative is serving us faithfully. Use your journal to write about how you realized your narrative might be a little troubled.

Direct message us YOUR story @Buddy_N_Soul on Instagram and be anonymously featured for a chance to **win a Buddy&Soul three month free membership.**

13 Lasting lessons from Acing the Fourth Trimester

Your fourth trimester may be coming to a close, but unlike Org Chem, you don't really leave what you've learned behind after the final. You're going to be a parent for the rest of your life, and how you do will affect your child for the rest of their lives (but no pressure, fam). So what are some of the lessons you've learned in the first few months of your baby's life, that will last long after your baby's sleeping the night, sporting a full set of teeth and yelling at you to knock before you come in, for God's sake? Be sure to add your own personal takeaway!

1. A 'good enough' mother is good enough. I'm not competing with Super Mom™ from Mommy&Me, I just need to be there for my baby.
2. There *is* no perfect mom. Super Mom™ may be putting on a perfect front, but there's no telling what aspects of parenthood she's struggling with behind closed doors.
3. Nutrition and exercise helps boost mood and self-esteem in your fourth trimester, and beyond.
4. Being a postnatal mom has its gifts and its challenges and that's okay. There's no rule that says you can't complain, and no rule that says you can't enjoy the good parts.
5. I may not be able control over how my baby acts and reacts; I can however, have control how I respond to my baby.
6. It's normal to feel overwhelmed; that doesn't mean I'm not doing it right!
7. Setting goals will help me feel motivated and that I'm doing something for myself.
8. Taking care of me is taking care of my baby.
9. Asking for help may make me vulnerable. It also allows me to get support.
10. Professionals are professionals because they know things I don't. Using them as resources can help.

Add some of your favorite lessons that you learned from this book:

11. ____

12. ____

13. ____

WHERE DO WE GO FROM HERE?

You've finished the Acing the Fourth Trimester book, but you haven't finished the journey. It doesn't end, it just gets better. Revisit this book, carry its ideas with you. Check out BuddynSoul.com and the rest of our books for all we have to offer. Spread the word. And change your life for good.

Loving Your Pregnant Body

Pregnancy can feel like an alien invasion right inside your body! If you're finding it challenging to come to terms with some of the changes your body is going through, welcome to the club. In this book, you'll find helpful, research-based actions you can take to keep your self-esteem up and your unfounded expectations down this pregnancy, no matter what changes your body is going through.

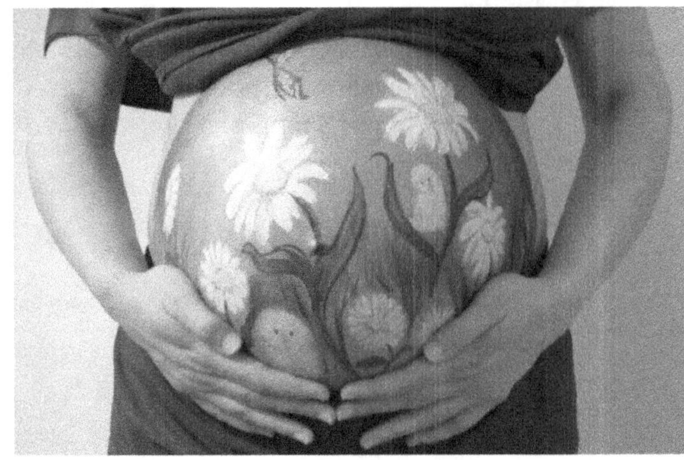

Goals you can achieve by reading 'Loving your Pregnant Body':

1. Accept your body regardless of its changes.
2. Let go of critical thoughts, fears, and unrealistic expectations around your pregnant body.
3. Appreciate the changes in your body as a part of the miracle of creating a new life.

Relationship Saver During Pregnancy

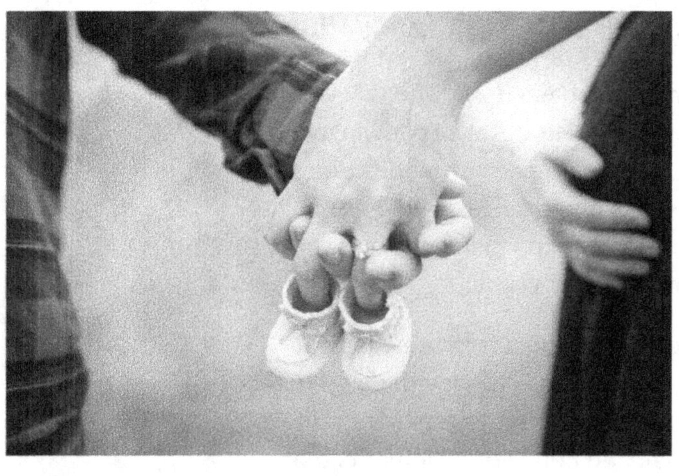

Pregnancy can put a strain on even the best relationships. That's why it's so important to preemptively support your relationship now, so your new family can be built on rock-solid foundations. Keeping in mind your needs, your partner's needs, and the needs of your relationship, this course will give you the know-how to strengthen your connection during pregnancy and beyond.

<u>Goals you can achieve by reading 'Relationship Saver During Pregnancy'</u>:

1. Identify your needs – both as two individuals and as a pair – as you navigate this pregnancy.
2. Strengthen your communication and build your connection with your partner.
3. Take responsibility for improving your relationship during pregnancy and beyond.

Sticking to Your Pregnancy Plan

You're having a baby (yay!) and you want everything to go smoothly. Following your doctor's orders concerning medication, vitamins, lifestyle changes, and diet is an important part of the plan...but that sure as heck ain't to say it's easy.

This book offers you a fresh new look at sticking to your medical provider's prenatal "rules." We'll explore the cognitive, emotional, and behavioral elements that can help you improve your health outcomes, and of course, your baby's.

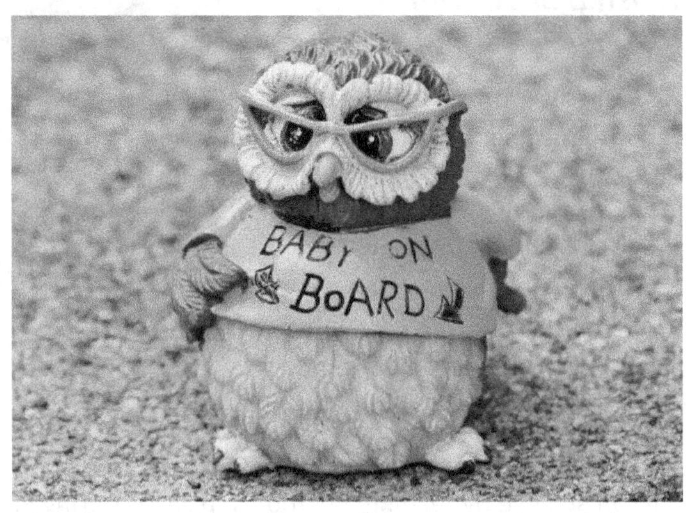

Goals you can achieve by reading 'Sticking to Your Pregnancy Plan':

1. Assume responsibility for sticking to your pregnancy health regimen.
2. Delve deeply into what may be holding you back from properly adhering to a healthy pregnant lifestyle.
3. Implement practical, research-based tools to help improve your adherence to your pregnancy plan.

WANT TO LEARN MORE? CHECK THESE OUT!

MOVIES

Three Men and a Baby (1987)

This comedy is about a man suddenly forced to take full responsibility for his baby daughter – a baby he never knew existed. The film appeals to anyone who has ever had a baby to care for, and will keep you rolling in laughter as you watch three men try to manage what often find yourself dealing with on your own.

Life as We Know it (2010)

When a little girl's parents die suddenly, her two godparents step in to raise her in their place. They face many struggles new parents do – needing to find the balance of putting their separate lives on hold, learning how to care for a new baby, and beginning to identify as a parent in addition to their other identities. This movie will make you laugh, and cry, and identify with the transition of becoming a parent.

MORE VIDEOS

Priscilla Dunstan on Oprah

Watch this fascinating clip to learn how your newborn baby makes distinct sounds when hungry, tired, uncomfortable, or in need of a burp. Learning about the ways your baby communicates with you will give you a new sense of control and allow you to overcome some of the feelings of helplessness that have overwhelmed you since the baby was born.

How motherhood supercharged my career: Gesine Thomson at TEDxOrangeCoast

Listen to an amazing, successful architect talk about how inspiring the challenges of motherhood were for her. How her experiences as a mother affected the way she worked with her colleagues, how she approached obstacles, and how she has always tried to add the magic of childhood into the projects she plans for adults.

RECOMMENDED APPS

Total Baby

This app helps you keep organized and sane regarding your baby. Use this attractive, fun app to track every aspect of your baby's care and development: immunizations, doctor visits, childhood illnesses, growth, feeding schedules, developmental milestones, and more.

Whenever you are feeling particularly lonely or down, use this app to keep you on track with regard to postpartum diet and weight loss, caring for your newborn, and dealing with baby blues. Use the postpartum depression test to monitor your emotional state and know if you need to seek outside help.

BOOKS

What to Expect First Year, by Heidi Murkoff and Sharon Mazel

Every new parent should own a copy of this best-selling guide to caring for you and your baby during the first year. Physical and mental health topics are discussed, as well as the kind of care and nurturing your baby needs as he or she grows and develops.

Better than Before: Mastering the Habits of our Everyday Lives, by Gretchen Rubin

Take your mind of your body and life, both of which feel like they might be falling apart, for a while, and just enjoy resting with your baby and reading this interesting book. Learn how to identify any bad or unproductive habits you may have, and how you can change your habits to improve your quality of life.

GADGETS AND PRODUCTS

Letters to My Baby: Write Now. Read Later. Treasure Forever.

This book of 12-fold-and-mail letters invites mothers to capture the fleeting memories of their babies' first years. Each letter bears a prompt for moms to reflect on their hopes and dreams for their little ones. The letters can be postdated, sealed up, and gifted for the years to come. In the future, their children get to break the seals to receive the greatest gift imaginable: a tangible expression of their mother's love. This heirloom-quality keepsake makes a priceless gift for the expectant or the more experienced mother.

Mom Life: A Snarky Adult Coloring Book (Humorous Coloring Books For Grown- Ups)

It's 6:30 PM. By some miracle, one of your kids is asleep while the other is watching cartoons in a food coma. Quick! Here's your chance! Grab some colored pencils and markers, this coloring book, and run to the bathroom (don't forget the wine)! First, lock the door and enjoy the solitude of private urination. Second, gulp down that wine and enjoy the most relaxing five minutes of your day as you surrender to the quietness and creativity of coloring. Celebrate the humor and frustration that are the highs and lows of motherhood featured in the pages of this book...... Happy Coloring!